Oh Crap! My Wife Has Breast Cancer

Nick Cox

Published by Nick Cox, 2024.

OH CRAP! MY WIFE HAS BREAST CANCER

First edition. July 28, 2024.

Copyright © 2024 Nick Cox.

ISBN: 979-8227943781

Written by Nick Cox.

Table of Contents

To my beautiful wife, Cayla, whose bravery and courage have been a constant source of strength and inspiration. This book is dedicated to you.

Preface

My journey alongside my wife, Cayla, who was diagnosed with stage 3 breast cancer, has led to profound changes and realizations. From handling the stress of her illness to finding new ways to support others, I've learned invaluable lessons. This book details my personal growth and the strategies I've developed to turn our experiences into a source of strength and inspiration for others.

A Sad Story

One of the most heartbreaking stories I encountered was at a fundraiser event for cancer patients hosted by a wonderful organization called Wiggin' Out, where Cayla was also a speaker. The founder of the organization shared how she became inspired to start the non-profit. She recounted a story about her childhood best friend, who was diagnosed with breast cancer as an adult. As soon as her friend became sick, her husband left her, stating he couldn't deal with a sick wife. He abandoned her, and she wound up in poverty and eventually died. I don't think I've heard a more gut-wrenching and convicting story in a long while.

This story hit home on so many levels. When Cayla was first diagnosed, some people commented that if Cayla were married to anyone else, they would be worried, but they knew I would stick by her. I didn't think much of it at the time, but after hearing the founder's story, I couldn't stop thinking about those earlier comments. How does someone make the decision to leave their spouse during such a critical time? The thought kept nagging at me, and I started to explore the reasons behind such actions.

I came to the conclusion that there are several reasons why men might leave their wives in these situations. The obvious explanation is that some men are selfish and were in the marriage for the wrong reasons. But there might be more to it—some men's fight-or-flight instincts might kick in, causing them to feel overwhelmed and unable to cope. Once that bridge is burned, I suppose there's no turning back.

This realization made me wonder if I could do something to save some of these marriages. Could I help build a community and alleviate the sense of overwhelm by sharing our story? This thought process ultimately led me to write this book.

By sharing our experiences, I hope to provide support and guidance to others navigating similar journeys. Saving marriages by promoting a long-term perspective has become a central mission. By encouraging open discussions about trauma and supporting one another, we can heal and grow. This book is part of my effort to fill that gap and provide the support that is so desperately needed.

Creative Outreach and Personal Growth

I'm writing this book to begin our outreach and share our experiences. This book serves as a comprehensive guide for husbands navigating their wives' cancer journeys, filled with practical advice, emotional support, and real-life stories. Writing it has allowed me to reflect deeply on our journey, organize our experiences, and present them in a way that can help others. The book is not just about telling our story but also about providing a roadmap for others who may feel lost and overwhelmed. My goal is to offer a resource that can be referred to at any stage of the cancer journey, providing comfort and guidance when it's needed most.

Cayla and I both have a YouTube channel where we share personal stories, offer advice, and connect with people from all over the world who are navigating the complexities of cancer. Through video content, we address common concerns, provide updates on Cayla's progress, and share tips on how to support a loved one through cancer. The visual and interactive nature of the channel allows for a more personal connection, making the advice and support feel more immediate and relatable.

In addition to the book and YouTube channel, I aim to establish a community space for husbands to talk and share their experiences. This community space, whether it's an online forum, a support group, or local meetups, will offer a safe and supportive environment where men can express their fears, frustrations, and triumphs without judgment. It's a place where they can find solidarity and support from others who understand what they're going through. Sharing experiences and advice will help alleviate the sense of isolation that many husbands feel and provide practical solutions to common problems.

Saving marriages by promoting a long-term perspective has become a central mission. It's about helping couples see beyond the immediate crisis and understand that their relationship can emerge stronger on the other side. By encouraging open discussions about trauma and supporting one another, we can heal and grow together. This means addressing not only the physical and medical aspects of cancer but also the emotional and psychological impact it has on relationships. Through future workshops, counseling, and open dialogue, couples can learn to communicate more effectively, support each other better, and rebuild their lives together.

By fostering a community of understanding and support, we aim to create a network where no one has to face these challenges alone. The combination of the book, the YouTube channel, and the community space provides a multifaceted approach to helping families navigate the complexities of cancer. Through these efforts, we hope to make a meaningful difference in the lives of those affected by this disease, offering them hope, support, and a path forward.

Introduction

Life has a way of throwing us curveballs when we least expect them. For me, that curveball came in the form of my wife Cayla's breast cancer diagnosis. It was a day that forever changed our lives and set us on a journey filled with fear, hope, pain, and resilience. As the newly elected mayor of our hometown, I was already grappling with the challenges of public office. Adding the role of caregiver to my responsibilities was overwhelming, to say the least.

This book, "Oh Crap, My Wife Has Breast Cancer," is a candid account of our family's journey through the trials and tribulations of battling cancer. It is a story of raw emotions, tough decisions, and the rollercoaster of experiences that come with a life-altering diagnosis. More importantly, it is a guide for other husbands, fathers, and families who find themselves in similar situations.

Throughout this book, I share our personal stories, the highs and lows, the moments of triumph and despair. From the initial shock of the diagnosis to the intricacies of treatment, from maintaining a semblance of normalcy for our children to dealing with the awkward and often painful realities of cancer, we faced it all. My goal is to provide practical advice, emotional support, and a sense of camaraderie for those navigating this difficult path.

I never imagined I would write a book like this, but I felt a calling to share our experiences in the hope that it might help others. Cancer is a battle fought not just by the patient but by their entire support system.

As husbands and caregivers, we need to be the pillars of strength for our wives, even when we feel like crumbling inside. This book is about learning to bend but not break, to find light in the darkest of times, and to emerge stronger on the other side.

Thank you for joining us on this journey. I hope our story provides you with the insights, strength, and comfort you need to face your own challenges.

Sincerely,

Nick Cox

Chapter 1: Oh Crap, This is Real

Life, with its capricious twists, often delivers blows we least expect. For us, it wasn't a singular event but the somber news that altered our very existence. I had just been elected Mayor of my hometown, poised for a future full of promise, when the announcement of Cayla's cancer brought everything to a halt before I even took office.

Cayla, my steadfast partner and source of strength, had been experiencing a persistent pain under her arm. Ever the embodiment of grace and resilience, she bore it quietly, though the discomfort lingered. We speculated on the cause—perhaps a strained muscle. With life's constant demands, I dismissed it as likely nothing serious.

We scheduled an appointment with Cayla's doctor, and life carried on as usual. Amidst our routines, we planned a much-needed family trip to Branson, Missouri, for some camping and relaxation. Branson, with its inviting outdoors, was a familiar refuge. It was during this trip, in the confined space of our camper shower, that Cayla discovered a lump in her breast. This discovery changed everything.

The realization struck hard. Panic surged, and overwhelming waves of grief engulfed me. The picturesque scenery of Branson, with its lush forests and serene lakes, suddenly felt like a cruel contrast to the turmoil within me. As we sat by the campfire that night, the crackling flames mirrored the anxiety burning in my chest.

Cayla and I, in our second marriages, had found a profound connection, a testament to our belief in soul mates. We had been married for nine years and cherished every moment together. Knowing how different and special this relationship was, compared to our previous marriages, made the thought of losing her unbearable. Memories of our first date and wedding day flooded my mind, now feeling like fragile treasures threatened by an uncertain future.

I remember thinking, "My God, my life is so good. I'm so happy to have found the person my soul loves, as the greeting cards say. How poetically terrible, how ironic, how dreadful that I might lose my wife. How will I survive as a widower? This is my luck. I'm cursed. No one should be this happy." I spiraled into despair.

In those moments, I reached out to a friend who had faced breast cancer the previous year. She offered perspective, explaining that often these things turn out to be false alarms. Reassured somewhat, I told myself repeatedly, "It's probably nothing," though doubt lingered at the edges of my mind.

Returning from our trip, we faced Cayla's doctor appointment. The clinic's sterile environment, with its antiseptic smell and harsh lighting, heightened our unease. The doctor immediately ordered an ultrasound. The technician, an old acquaintance of Cayla's, struggled to maintain her composure. The radiologist noted a high probability of cancer and recommended a biopsy. This news was a heavy blow, but we pressed on.

When your medical staff is upset, it is unnerving. In our small city, everyone knows everyone. While we appreciated the love shown by the medical staff, it didn't inspire optimism.

The next few days were a blur. We tried to maintain normalcy, but the looming appointment weighed heavily on us. The day before my swearing-in ceremony, we received the biopsy results. Sitting in the waiting room, the ticking clock amplified our tension. When the surgeon finally called us in, her somber expression conveyed the gravity of the situation.

"We need to talk about the results," she began. "The biopsy confirmed it's breast cancer. It's the textbook nasty kind." This term, "textbook nasty," would become all too familiar in our journey.

Time seemed to freeze. The world faded as I processed the words: breast cancer. My thoughts raced—Cayla, the children, our life together. I had a city to run, responsibilities to meet. How would we navigate this?

Leaving the doctor's office, the diagnosis weighed heavily on us. We drove home in silence, lost in thought. That night, as we lay in bed, Cayla whispered, "Nick, what are we going to do?" I took her hand, feeling its warmth and strength. "We're going to take it one day at a time," I replied, trying to reassure both of us.

The next day, as Cayla held the Bible and I took the oath of office, I thought as I stood there repeating my oath "How am I going to get through this and run an entire city at the same time?" The weight of the world seemed on my shoulders, and no one in the public knew what we were facing as a family.

One of the hardest parts was telling our children. They were teenagers, preoccupied with sports, school, friends, and their significant others. They needed to understand what was happening. We gathered them in the living room, searching for the right words.

"Kids, we need to talk about something important," I began, my voice trembling. "Cayla is sick. She has breast cancer. The next year will be hard, but her medical team has a plan, and we will get through this together."

Their faces reflected shock and confusion. We answered their questions honestly, reassuring them of our determination to face this as a family. Surprisingly, they accepted the news better than I anticipated. Perhaps their teenage preoccupations shielded them from the full weight of the situation. As we hugged them, I felt a renewed resolve.

The following days were a whirlwind. We informed close friends and family, seeking support and prayers. Each conversation was emotionally draining but reminded us of the strong network surrounding us. We shared our journey on social media, keeping everyone informed and gathering support. Weekly updates on Facebook detailed our ups and downs, the outpouring of love and encouragement strengthening us. The first post read: "'You have breast cancer'—words we never wanted to hear and didn't foresee for 2023. Please pray for Cayla Cox and our family as we spend this year getting her cancer-free. She starts Tuesday with 24 weeks of chemo. We are thankful and blessed to be surrounded by prayer warriors and caring people. Our hope is in the Lord."

We soon met with the oncologist, Dr. Peddi, to discuss the treatment plan. We were eager to understand the steps ahead. The anticipation was nerve-wracking, but having a plan was a relief. Dr. Peddi laid out an aggressive plan: chemotherapy, surgery, and radiation. It seemed an endless road, but he assured us it was the best course given the cancer's stage and aggressiveness. "We have a tough journey ahead," he said, "but we will fight this together."

Given Cayla's age of 36, the battle plan was straightforward yet intense. The strategy was to administer the strongest treatments possible to ensure maximum effectiveness. "We are going to hold nothing back," Dr. Peddi affirmed.

I remember sitting in that sterile, cold office, listening as the doctor explained the side effects of chemotherapy: hair loss, nausea, fatigue, and numerous other potential issues. It was overwhelming. Cayla squeezed my hand, and in her eyes, I saw determination. She was ready to fight, no matter the battle's ferocity.

Amid our personal turmoil, our community's support became our beacon. The people of Minden rallied around us with unwavering support—meals appeared on our doorstep, offers to help with the kids poured in, and messages of love, prayers, and encouragement flooded our inboxes. Each act of kindness reminded us that we were not alone in this battle.

The day of Cayla's first chemotherapy session was fraught with anxiety and dread. Arriving at the hospital early, we navigated the maze-like hallways to the oncology department. The chemo room, stark and clinical, was filled with reclining chairs, loud TVs, and IV stands. The sight of other patients, each with their own story of struggle, was both humbling and sobering.

The chemotherapy process was different from what I had imagined. It was highly organized, and we quickly fell into a routine. The image of cattle being led to slaughter crossed my mind frequently. "Mrs. Cox, you will start on the 2nd floor for lab work, then proceed to the 3rd floor to discuss the results with your oncologist. Finally, back down to the 2nd floor for chemo administration."

Most cancer patients at our hospital attended an orientation called Chemo 100 or 101, but we skipped this as the doctors insisted there was no time to waste. I sat by Cayla's side, holding her hand as the nurse inserted the IV. The first drop of toxic medicine began to flow, and a surge of emotion overwhelmed me. This was real. This was happening.

As the chemotherapy drugs entered her bloodstream, each session lasted several hours. We would talk, read, or sit in silence, drawing strength from each other's presence. The world seemed to slow down, minutes stretched into hours, and every second felt like an eternity. It was as if we were trapped in a tunnel with no light at the end.

Our faith and the incredible support from our community were crucial in those early days. We were very public on social media about Cayla's diagnosis. I believe we were on every prayer list within a hundred miles or more. A friend, a local attorney, remarked, "If God responds to the number of people praying, Cayla is going to get that blessing."

Cayla and I became each other's pillars of strength. There were days when the weight of it all felt unbearable, but we learned to lean on each other. We cried together, laughed together, and found solace in each other's presence. Our love grew stronger, forged in the fire of adversity. The bond we shared, tested and tempered by our trials, became an unbreakable source of support.

One evening, Cayla turned to me and said, "Nick, we're going to get through this. One day at a time." Her words became our mantra. We took it day by day, focusing on small victories and holding on to hope for a brighter future. Each day that passed without major setbacks was a triumph, a testament to our resilience and determination.

The journey had just begun, but in those early days, we learned the importance of support, faith, and resilience. We discovered a strength within us that we never knew we had. And through it all, we held on to hope, knowing that together, we could face whatever came our way. The path ahead was uncertain, but we were ready to navigate it with unwavering resolve.

Our story was only starting to unfold, and the road ahead was long and uncertain. But we faced it with newfound determination and unwavering belief in each other. This was just the beginning of our battle, and we were ready to fight with everything we had.

Key Points to Remember During This Time

- ***Take it One Day at a Time:*** The road ahead can seem overwhelming if you try to see too far into the distance. Focus on each day as it comes, tackling the details, treatments, medicines, and decisions step by step.

- ***Kids Are Tougher Than You Think:*** Children often possess a resilience that surprises us. Keep the lines of communication open, speaking honestly and frequently, for it's easy to overlook their need for information and reassurance.

- ***Lean on Your Support System:*** Do not hesitate to draw upon the strength of friends, family, and community. Their support can provide much-needed solace and encouragement.

- ***Breast Cancer is Not a Death Sentence***: Remember, nothing has fundamentally changed at the moment of diagnosis except your awareness of what her body already knew. Maintain your composure and calm.

- ***The Path Forward is a Journey, Not an Overnight Fix:*** This process will take time and perseverance. Understand that the journey is long, and patience will be your steadfast companion.

- ***It Changes Your World, But It's Not the End of the World:*** While this diagnosis will alter your life, it doesn't spell the end. Adapt and find new ways to move forward together, discovering strength in your unity.

Chapter 2: Oh Crap, Freak Out Phase

The journey into our nightmare began, as most do, with denial and a faint, desperate hope that "maybe it's nothing." For weeks, I clung to that hope, repeating it like a mantra, trying to will the universe into compliance. But slowly, inexorably, the truth emerged, bringing with it the full weight of dread. This was not just something; this was the thing I had feared most. The diagnosis was a "textbook nasty cancer." It was a phrase that carried the weight of a death sentence. There was no mistaking it; Cayla had cancer. At 39, I found myself staring down the biggest challenge of my life. I had faced my share of hardships before, including a painful, dramatic, and abrupt divorce, but this was different. This was a fight for survival, requiring a strength I wasn't sure I possessed.

When the oncologist delivered the news, my first reaction was sheer, unadulterated panic. As I mentioned earlier, the fear of losing Cayla tore at my very soul. In the quiet solitude of my private moments, I cried. The fear was a relentless tormentor, gnawing at me with every breath. I envisioned a future without her and felt the crushing weight of that possibility. How would I manage without her? How would I take care of our kids? Can I mentally manage being newly widowed and be the mayor? Our minds, in moments of crisis, conjure up the most outlandish scenarios. It's part of our nature, I suppose.

The oncologist, however, brought a glimmer of hope. He spoke of survival rates—90%, a figure that seemed like a lifeline thrown to a drowning man. This reassurance, coupled with the realization that many people I knew were breast cancer survivors, helped. These were individuals who had faced the beast and emerged victorious, some with one breast and a prosthetic, yet living full, vibrant lives. This knowledge was a relief to my tormented soul.

One story from this tumultuous period stands out. We had a dear friend, a woman of remarkable strength and grace, who was also battling breast cancer. In a private moment, we confided our fears about Cayla to her. This woman, often described as a Barbie doll for her perfect appearance, revealed, her bald head—a stark and humbling symbol of her struggle. She explained that her cancer was aggressive, requiring her to wear a monitor to regulate her hormones, a constant reminder of her ongoing battle. The monitor adjusted her hormone levels every 15 minutes, a relentless routine that kept her alive. I remember praying fervently that Cayla's case wouldn't be as severe. Our friend, ever compassionate, assured us that most cases weren't as dire as hers, offering a glimmer of hope.

When we made Cayla's diagnosis public, that same friend reached out to us. She tried to console me, explaining that her initial diagnosis had been very bad like Cayla's but had since improved. My fear for Cayla's life intensified. "You mean the lady that has the bad cancer is telling me that Cayla's cancer is worse. We are doomed!" The thought of losing her was a constant shadow, darkening even the brightest moments.

As a husband, father, and provider, my worries quickly turned to our household finances. I was transitioning to being mayor full-time, with plans for Cayla to run our business. During the campaign, I often reassured people that Cayla had everything under control. I had spent years preparing her for this transition, but life had other plans. I gathered my loyal employees and explained the situation, asking for their help. They stepped up, running the business with dedication. The city's insurance was also a real help, and I also discovered a small cancer policy I had bought years ago, which kept us afloat. If you're reading this and don't have a cancer policy, get one. It's invaluable.

After exhausting my financial freak-out, I turned to home remedies. In my quest for a feeling of some kind of control, I dove headfirst into research. I scoured the internet for information on cancer treatments, reading everything I could get my hands on. I watched countless videos, read dozens of books, and explored every possible avenue of treatment. I became obsessed with finding a solution, a way to fix what was broken. From alternative treatments like Joe Tippens' Fenbendazole remedy to Jane McLelland's "How to Starve Cancer," I explored them all. I looked into alkaline water, Celtic salts, no sugar diets, and natural hot springs. I made Cayla drink concoctions like baking soda water, hoping that one of these remedies would make a difference. It was a way for me to feel like I was doing something, anything, to help.

After that consoling call from our friend, I called my mom and cried like a baby. I made a deal with her: everyone expected me to be strong for Cayla, but I needed someone to lose my crap with. My mom, stoic but motherly, became my lifeline. She wasn't a worrier—that was my dad's specialty. We even nicknamed him Mr. Freakout many years ago for his great ability to worry enough for everyone. My mom was a rock, and surprisingly, I didn't need to call her often. For that, I'm proud—especially because I'm Mr. Freakout Jr., after all.

The days turned into weeks, and the weeks into months. Each day brought its own set of challenges and fears. I found myself moving on past the idea of death. Once I heard the 90% chance and the oncologist say "we are going to get rid of this damn cancer," I was good to go on that part.

As the weeks went by, I found a semblance of routine. The initial shock had worn off, and we settled into a new normal. Cayla began her treatments, and we adjusted our lives around the relentless schedule of doctor's appointments and hospital visits. I continued to juggle my responsibilities as mayor and business owner, finding solace in the familiar routines of work. But beneath the surface, one thing never went away: cancer, the textbook nasty kind. These words were ever-present, like a storm cloud on the horizon.

There's something about cancer that is all-consuming. It becomes the center of your world, the lens through which you view everything. Every decision, every action, is influenced by it. It's like the Willie Nelson song, "You Were Always on My Mind." Cancer was always on my mind, an ever-present specter that haunted our every moment.

Throughout this time, I clung to the small victories. The good days, when Cayla felt strong and hopeful, were like rays of sunshine breaking through the clouds. I cherished those moments, holding onto them as a lifeline. They were reminders that, despite everything, there was still hope. And hope, I found, was a powerful thing.

Key Points to Remember During This Time

- *Freaking out about death* is normal for a spouse of a newly diagnosed cancer patient. It's a fear that lurks in the back of your mind, ever-present and relentless. Acknowledge it, but don't let it consume you.

- *Freaking out about money* is also natural. Cancer is not just an emotional and physical burden; it's a financial one as well. Do what you can to prepare, but remember that there is help available. Don't be afraid to accept it.

- *Freaking out about home remedies* was a distraction for me. While some may not have helped, they didn't hurt either. The important thing was that they gave me a sense of control, however small. Also, you need to know that baking soda water tastes terrible.

- *Designate a person to be weak with* This was crucial for me. Having someone to confide in, someone who could bear the weight of my fears, made all the difference. For me, that person was my mom. Find your person and lean on them when you need to.

Chapter 3: Oh Crap, Daytime Mayor, Nighttime Caregiver

The day before I was sworn in as Mayor of Minden, Cayla and I received the results from her biopsy. The words "It is textbook breast cancer" echoed in our minds, but there was no time to fully process it. The next day, I stood before a crowd, with Cayla by my side, holding the Bible. As I took the oath of office, a mix of pride and fear consumed me. I remember thinking, how could I manage the responsibilities of running a city while my wife faced the battle of her life? How can I keep it together for the city when I'm falling apart inside? The ceremony was a blur of handshakes, smiles, and congratulations, but my mind was elsewhere, weighed down by the uncertainty of what lay ahead for our family.

Every day brought a new set of challenges. By day, I was Mayor Nick Cox, responsible for the wellbeing of Minden's residents. By night, I was Nick, the husband, and father, grappling with the harsh realities of Cayla's illness. It felt like I was living two lives, each demanding my full attention and emotional strength. The mornings started early with briefings and meetings, discussing city budgets, infrastructure projects, and community issues. My afternoons were filled with public appearances, ribbon cuttings, and addressing constituents' concerns. I had to be present, engaged, and responsive, all while a part of me was constantly worried about Cayla.

I quickly learned that compartmentalizing was essential. During office hours, I had to focus on city issues—addressing community needs, attending meetings, and making decisions that impacted the lives of my citizens. Running a city involves managing numerous departments and dealing with a vast array of issues. These responsibilities required attention, leadership, and strategy. Immersing myself in these tasks turned out to be a blessing in disguise. Being the newly elected mayor with so much on my shoulders and a wife newly diagnosed with cancer was not the bad fortune everyone thought it was. In many ways, it kept me sane. The volume of things I had to learn and tackle provided an escape from dwelling on cancer every minute of every day. Though cancer was always on my mind, the city's demands offered a necessary distraction from the emotional toll of our home life.

Yet, the moment I stepped out of City Hall, my mind would shift back to Cayla. Stepping out of the door felt like walking into a cloud that dimmed the sunshine, and I would start wondering how she was feeling, worrying about the next doctor's appointment, and wishing time would fast forward. My two-minute drive home often became a mental transition, preparing myself to switch roles from mayor to caregiver. I would arrive home to find Cayla exhausted from her treatments. The intensity of my day would shift from full speed ahead to a slow march toward bedtime.

Most of her chemo treatments left her completely wiped out, with no energy. She often slept all day, and we would go to bed by 8 pm. This routine, though depressing, was necessary for her recovery and a way for me to pass the days. Historically, Cayla and my favorite thing to do was to jump in a vehicle and go for a ride. We enjoyed exploring destinations we never planned to visit, simply spending time together. But that year, there were no travels, no day trips. I remember longing for normalcy and suggesting we go to one of our favorite places for lunch after a doctor's appointment. Cayla, always sweet, agreed, even though she wasn't feeling well. We sat down, ordered food, but before it arrived, she was totally out of it. I remember worrying the waitress might think I had drugged her. We got our food to go. That year, our camper never moved, and we didn't swim in our pool. These were the dark ages for us.

One of the biggest blessings during this time was the outpouring of support from our community. People I had never met reached out with words of encouragement, prayers, and offers to help. This collective kindness reminded me that even in my dual roles, I was not alone. Our neighbors, friends, and even strangers provided a network of support that buoyed us through the darkest days. I was constantly amazed by the generosity and compassion of those around us, and it reinforced my commitment to serve this incredible community.

The journey did not go as you might think or even as I might have guessed. Initially, I expected my response to be filled with weakness, pleading with God to change things, a stronger prayer life, or perhaps blaming God or myself. For the first few weeks, this was true. But after the initial shock, I took a different approach. To reference the Pink Floyd song, I became comfortably numb. This numbing wasn't intentional or planned; it just happened. Numb made me strong. It kept me solid during the challenges, mellow during the good times, and helped me ride through the storms without taking normal things too seriously. Numbness served me well as mayor. That first year set the precedent for my tenure, and maintaining a stoic demeanor helped me navigate the complexities of city administration. With 222 employees, it was easy to let emotions influence decisions, but my new survival skill of automatic numbness helped me stay focused and effective.

People often think that being stoic means you don't care, but it's quite the opposite. I cared deeply for my wife and my city. I realized that the best thing I could do for both was to remain a rock. A husband and wife's emotions often feed off each other, and for us, this proved true. If Cayla needed to be strong, then I had to be strong as well. This applied to the city, too. An organization takes on the personality of its leader.

Transparency became a crucial part of my leadership style. While I didn't divulge every detail of our personal struggles, I shared enough to let people know that I was navigating difficult situations. This honesty helped build trust with my constituents and brought an unexpected level of empathy and understanding from them. This openness fostered a deeper connection with the community, as people saw me not just as their mayor, but as a fellow human being facing real struggles. I remember one well-meaning lady telling Cayla that her having cancer made us seem more relatable, more normal.

Amidst the chaos, there were reminders that life, even in its toughest phases, still held beauty and joy. I gained a new appreciation for people during this time. At the start of our cancer journey, I was somewhat jaded towards the public, but every card, kind word, heartfelt Facebook post, meal brought to the house, and church prayer list showed me that people really care. I was touched by how many people, even those who barely knew us, called Cayla by name and said they were praying for her. It deepened my love for serving the community.

We celebrated small victories, like a good day after chemo or a shared laugh over a funny story. These moments were a balm to our spirits, helping us stay connected and hopeful. Looking back, this chapter of our lives taught me invaluable lessons about resilience, community, and the power of faith. Balancing my duties as mayor with the responsibilities of being a supportive husband was no easy feat, but it reinforced the importance of prioritizing what truly mattered. I learned to delegate more effectively at work, trusting my team to handle tasks I would have otherwise taken on myself. This not only lightened my load but also empowered my staff and improved the efficiency of our city government.

In the end, it wasn't about being perfect in either role. It was about showing up every day, doing the best I could, and leaning on the support of those around me. It was about finding strength in vulnerability and hope in the midst of uncertainty. Cayla's journey through cancer and my journey as mayor became intertwined, each experience shaping and informing the other. I emerged from this period with a deeper appreciation for life's fragility and a renewed commitment to serving my community with empathy and strength.

Key Points to Remember During This Time

- ***Compartmentalizing Roles:*** Effectively balancing the demands of a career and being a caregiver required compartmentalizing responsibilities, allowing focus on work issues during office hours and providing an emotional escape from personal challenges.

- ***Community Support:*** The outpouring of support from the community was invaluable, providing both emotional and practical assistance. This collective kindness highlighted the importance of community and the power of coming together during difficult times.

- ***Finding Strength in Numbness:*** Adopting a numb, stoic demeanor helped navigate the emotional and practical challenges of both roles. This approach allowed for effective decision-making and emotional resilience, proving that strength can be found in unexpected coping mechanisms.

- ***Transparency and Empathy:*** Being transparent about personal struggles helped build trust and empathy within the community. Sharing enough to let people understand the challenges fostered deeper connections and highlighted the humanity behind leadership.

Chapter 4: Oh Crap, I Forgot About the Kids

When Cayla was diagnosed with cancer, it wasn't just our lives as a couple that were upended; the entire family dynamic was thrown into chaos. Only later did I fully comprehend the impact on the children. My stoicism, which served me well in my professional life and as a devoted caregiving husband, proved inadequate for the role of a father.

During this period, the kids were essentially left to their own devices. By that, I mean completely on their own. Cayla, known to all as super mom, was the type who volunteered for every homecoming float, led children's church, and organized fall carnivals to ensure her kids had the best experiences possible. If Cayla had three pieces of pizza left, those would go to the kids while she went without, smiling all the while. Her love language is giving, a caretaker by nature. But for the first time, this selfless attention was not available to them.

Cayla had one job during this tumultuous time—getting through cancer. This singular focus was all she could physically and mentally manage.

I suspect that part of the kids being somewhat overlooked was due to their age. Whether the boys were too absorbed in their own adolescent concerns to notice Cayla's struggles, or lacked the emotional maturity to express their feelings, they seemed okay on the surface. This did not demand my attention. Remember, I was working all day and in bed by

8 pm. My primary responsibility was being with Cayla, leaving the kids largely to fend for themselves.

My determination to forge ahead through the challenges meant I lacked the emotional bandwidth to support them. This approach permeated all aspects of my life, blinding me to the impact on my children. Alleigh, my stepdaughter, was particularly affected. Despite being my stepdaughter, we were very close. I married Cayla when Alleigh had just turned six years old, and out of all three kids, her personality most closely mirrors mine.

Throughout Cayla's year-long battle, Alleigh was a real rockstar. During her last years in high school, a time when most kids focus on their future and enjoy their final school experiences, Alleigh took on the responsibility of managing household chores. She washed dishes, swept and mopped floors, and kept the house in order. Meanwhile, I was cold and harsh, my stoicism amplifying these traits. I did not realize the extent of my behavior until nearly the end of Cayla's treatment.

One night, Alleigh broke down. She told me she was giving everything she had to help us through this incredibly difficult time. She serves others by doing chores, a reflection of her way of coping and showing love. Her breakdown was a wake-up call for me. Alleigh, who appeared so tough on the outside, was actually very tender on the inside. She confessed that her emotions were not being supported and that she missed the old Nick—the jolly and happy Nick she once knew. Her words struck a deep chord. She was right. Nothing about me was happy or jolly. I was stoic and, in truth, likely very depressed.

Meanwhile, my son Noah and my stepson Garrett, both in their first couple of years in high school and only a month apart in age, seemed less affected. They were thick as thieves, always together, and didn't seem to worry about much. But just because they didn't show it didn't mean they weren't affected. I later realized I needed to be more attentive to all my children, recognizing that each coped with the situation in their own ways.

Reflecting on this period, I understood the importance of honest communication with the kids about the situation. It's crucial to explain the diagnosis, treatment, and changes in family dynamics in a way they can understand. Involving them in the journey without overwhelming them is key to helping them cope.

Balancing attention between caring for a spouse and supporting the children, even teenagers, is challenging. Effective strategies to divide time and attention are necessary. Involving other family members or friends to provide additional support can ease the burden. Importantly, self-care for the caregiver is crucial to be present and effective for both the spouse and the children.

This experience taught me the importance of being mindful of my children's needs during such a difficult journey. Being a strong and dedicated husband did not excuse me from being an emotionally available father. It's a hard lesson, but one that ultimately brought our family closer and helped me grow as a parent.

The stoic demeanor I adopted during this time was a sincere and natural coping mechanism, but it also created distance between me and my children. Alleigh's brave and heartfelt confrontation was a turning point. Her ability to articulate her feelings and needs opened my eyes to the emotional void I had left in her life. Her resilience and strength were remarkable, yet it underscored the need for emotional support and connection that every child deserves, especially in times of family crisis.

Noah and Garrett's seemingly unaffected demeanor was deceptive. Teenagers often mask their true feelings, and my initial interpretation of their behavior was misguided. They, too, needed their father's attention, even if they didn't outwardly show it. It's a reminder that all children, regardless of their outward behavior, need reassurance, support, and understanding from their parents.

Moving forward, I committed to being more present for my kids, to listen more, and to engage with them on an emotional level. It's about finding that balance—being there for your spouse while also being there for your children. The experience with Cayla's cancer was a harsh but valuable teacher. It taught me the importance of self-awareness and the need to continually work on being the best parent I can be, even in the face of overwhelming challenges.

In the end, we all emerged stronger, having navigated this incredibly tough journey together. The bonds with my children grew deeper as I learned to be more present and attentive to their needs. This chapter of our lives, though painful and challenging, was also a period of significant growth and understanding. It reinforced the importance of family, the power of communication, and the necessity of balancing all roles with compassion and love.

Key Points to Remember During This Time

- ***Balancing Roles is Essential:*** It's crucial to find a balance between being a supportive spouse and an attentive parent, even during challenging times like a family health crisis.
- ***Emotional Availability Matters:*** Being emotionally available to your children is just as important as being a dedicated caregiver. Kids need reassurance and support, especially when a parent is seriously ill.
- ***Open Communication is Key:*** Honest and age-appropriate communication with children about the family's situation helps them cope and feel included, reducing their feelings of being overlooked.
- ***Self-awareness and Growth:*** Recognizing and addressing one's emotional shortcomings can lead to personal growth and stronger family bonds. Being self-aware and willing to change can positively impact the entire family's well-being.

Chapter 5: Oh Crap, More Cake

Let me take you on a journey deep into the heart of Louisiana, where tradition runs as deep as the Mississippi River and the king cake reigns supreme. Picture, if you will, a grand, circular confection, braided with the skill of an artisan and baked to golden perfection. This is no ordinary cake; it is adorned with the vibrant hues of Mardi Gras—purple, green, and gold. Hidden within its sweet, doughy depths lies a small plastic baby, a symbol of good fortune and a promise of celebration to come.

When the word spread about Cayla's diagnosis, the outpouring of support from our community was as abundant and heartfelt as the spring floods. Friends and neighbors, in an effort to offer comfort and solidarity, showered us with an unending stream of desserts. We had homemade pies, cakes, brownies, but my biggest weakness was king cakes. And we had every version of king cake you could get your hands on. Our kitchen became a repository of sugary goodwill, each dessert a testament to the love and concern of those around us.

The arrival of each cake was both a blessing and a challenge. Initially, we welcomed these offerings with open arms, grateful for the sweet distraction from the harsh realities we were facing. But as the days turned into weeks, the sheer volume of cakes became almost comical. Our home now bore a striking resemblance to a bustling bakery during carnival season.

One evening, after a particularly grueling day at the hospital, we returned home, bone-weary and emotionally spent. As we walked through the door, the familiar sweet scent hit us immediately. There, sitting proudly on the kitchen counter, was yet another king cake, its sugar-dusted surface gleaming like a beacon of comfort. Despite her exhaustion, Cayla managed to muster a twinkle in her eye. With a wry smile, she turned to me and said, "Nick, if you keep eating these king cakes, they'll have to widen the door to your office."

Her words, infused with humor and resilience, brought much-needed laughter to our home. The cakes, in all their sugary splendor, had become more than just desserts. They were symbols of the community's unwavering support, each slice a tangible reminder that we were not alone in this fight.

This chapter of my life was filled with constant nagging stress, and at home, there wasn't much excitement happening. I found a lot of comfort in these desserts, especially the king cakes. I remember at one of Cayla's oncologist visits, the doctor told her that she needed to focus all her energy on getting better and not worry about dieting. He went on to say, "This is no time to worry about losing weight." So I would joke with people and say the doctor said, "This is not the time to lose weight." Yes, I know he wasn't talking about me, but it helped me enjoy the king cakes, pies, and brownies every evening! And the pounds were sneaking up on me like a gator in the bayou. We joked that soon we'd need to add a gym membership to our list of medical expenses. The weight gain was a physical manifestation of the stress and comfort-seeking that marked this chapter of our lives.

In the midst of all this, we learned a crucial lesson about the importance of accepting help from others. I was totally against a Meal Train in the beginning. I think my pride and ego were not ready to be humbled like that. I reluctantly agreed to a friend setting us up a meal train, and the first week of having it, Cayla was admitted to the hospital, 40 minutes away from our house. I remember thinking, I've got to arrange for dinner for the kids, then it hit me that a loved one was bringing over a meal that night. What a relief. I learned that during these times, it's great to let people love on you, and where we come from, people show love by bringing meals.

It's not always easy to accept help, especially when you're used to being the one offering it. But in times of crisis, letting others in and accepting their support can make all the difference. The meals were more than just food; they were a lifeline. They reminded us that our community was standing with us, ready to lift us up when we felt we couldn't stand on our own.

Accepting help is an act of courage and humility. It allowed us to conserve our energy for the battles that truly mattered. It also gave our friends and neighbors a way to express their care and concern, creating a web of support that was both strong and deeply comforting. There is a life lesson I needed to learn, and that is being able to receive.

In the spirit of generosity, and in an effort to manage our expanding waistlines, we began sharing the bounty. We distributed slices of cake to our friends, family, coworkers, Cayla's medical team, and anyone else who might benefit from a little sweetness in their day. This act of sharing became a way to stay connected and give back to the community that had shown us such overwhelming kindness.

The "cake phase" of our journey, marked by an abundance of baked goods and a few extra pounds, was an unexpected yet heartwarming chapter. It taught us the importance of balance, the power of humor in the face of adversity, and the profound impact of accepting help from others. And now, whenever I see a king cake, I am reminded of those days, filled with gratitude for the love and laughter that helped us through.

Key Points to Remember During This Time

- ***Embrace Community Support:*** People want to help you, and bringing food is often the best way they know how. Accepting help from friends, neighbors, and the community provides essential relief and comfort. Allow others to show their love and support, and don't hesitate to lean on them when needed.
- ***Find Humor and Balance:*** Use humor to lighten the emotional load and maintain perspective.
- ***Share Generosity and Express Gratitude:*** When blessed with an abundance, share with others to spread kindness and maintain community spirit.
- ***Pick Your Battles:*** In a time when your home mimics a nursing home, if a slice of king cake brings a little joy, then eat that king cake! This is a season to get away with being fat and happy!

Chapter 6: Oh Crap, This is Awkward

Cancer, in its relentless progression, doesn't just affect the body; it intrudes into every corner of life, turning even the simplest moments into awkward challenges. It's like an uninvited guest who barges in and upends your entire household, refusing to leave. This chapter recounts the deeply personal and often uncomfortable experiences Cayla and I faced during her treatment. These moments tested our resolve and reshaped our understanding of normalcy. By sharing them, I hope to provide comfort and insight for others navigating a similar path.

People's Comments and Advice

One of the most trying aspects was dealing with people. Everyone has an opinion during a crisis, and they feel compelled to share it. We received a litany of unsolicited advice, from alternative treatments to miracle diets. "Have you tried juicing?" or "My friend took this miracle supplement and was cured!" These comments, though well-meaning, often felt dismissive of Cayla's condition. We quickly learned to smile, nod, and filter out the noise.

One person suggested we try a specific herbal remedy, assuring us it had cured their cousin's friend. Another insisted that alkaline water was the secret to beating cancer and went as far as bringing us a case of it. Then there was the suggestion to avoid all sugar because "cancer feeds on sugar." While we appreciated the concern, these pieces of advice often added to the stress and confusion we were already facing.

Some folks seemed to think they had the right to comment on our decisions or speculate about our future. Remarks like, "You should stay positive," or "Everything happens for a reason," felt like empty platitudes that minimized our pain. Navigating these conversations without offending those who genuinely cared but didn't fully understand our reality was a delicate dance.

Friendships in waiting rooms were another unexpected aspect. Radiation treatments meant regular visits, and we often saw the same faces. We formed connections, sharing stories and experiences. These friendships could be comforting, providing a sense of camaraderie. However, they could also be awkward, especially when we were not in the mood to socialize but felt obligated to engage with those around us. These interactions often required a delicate balance between being friendly and maintaining personal boundaries.

Hair Loss and Regrowth

Losing hair was a significant and visible part of the journey. Watching Cayla lose her hair was heartbreaking. Two weeks after she started chemotherapy, we knew her hair was going to fall out. To take control of the inevitable, we sat Cayla down in the living room, gathered the kids, and shaved her head. I've done many hard things in my life, but shaving Cayla's head was among the toughest. Tears streamed down my face as I did it. The kids were there, and I wasn't prepared for my emotional response.

Cayla's appearance was a high priority for her. She loved having her hair done, dyed, and often wore extensions. She adored long eyelashes and even had her eyebrows tattooed for prominence. Chemo was about to take all of that away. It wasn't just the hair on her head; she lost her eyebrows, eyelashes, and body hair. This drastic change was tough to handle emotionally. Hair has such a strong connection to identity, and losing it can feel like losing a part of oneself. The process of shaving her head was a poignant moment for us, filled with tears and reluctant acceptance.

The stages of regrowth were equally awkward. Her hair grew back different in texture and color, making her look and feel different. She was very excited about the sprouts of new hair. It was a sign of a new beginning. There were days she hated the sight of herself in the mirror, and all I could do was remind her how beautiful she was to me. We purchased wigs early on, but she rarely wore them. It just wasn't the same. Cayla was proud to rock her bald head, and her bravery with the people she encountered will never be forgotten. Each stage of regrowth brought new challenges.

Challenges with Sexual Intimacy

Cancer treatments wreak havoc on the body in numerous ways, and one of the most personal areas affected is sexual intimacy. The treatments left Cayla feeling sick, tired, and unattractive.

Another thing that no one warned us about was the toxicity of the medications. One type of chemotherapy made her poisonous to me. Imagine that—a treatment saving her life was so toxic that one kiss could poison me! There was even a discussion about whether I should sleep in the same bed as her. It was a mind-blowing process.

A spouse should also be prepared for a complete lack of desire on her part, which takes a toll on intimacy. Cancer robbed me of all the cosmetic things my wife had going for her. She didn't have the energy, health, or desire for intimacy. I didn't know when it would ever return. It's a hard thing to deal with.

Our relationship dynamic shifted significantly during this time. I had to learn to be patient and understanding, recognizing that physical intimacy wasn't always possible. At least not in the ways we traditionally would. We explored other ways to stay connected like holding hands and expressing our love through words and actions rather than physical touch. The soul that I love so deeply was still there, despite being tattered and weary. I could endure this period and look forward to rebuilding back to where we were before cancer, but at the same time, I know nothing will ever be the same. It was a difficult adjustment, but finding new ways to be intimate helped us maintain our bond.

Interacting with Medical Staff

Medical staff interactions were another source of awkwardness. Our oncologist was fantastic, but the first thing he would do was examine her breast. That takes some getting used to. Cayla had to get used to being exposed and touched frequently by doctors and nurses.

They also led off with questions like, "How are you feeling? Do you have diarrhea? How runny was it? What color? How powerful?" Nothing tosses off the cloak of dignity like medical issues. The very fact that when you go into the hospital, you have to wear a gown with no backside coverage is a testament to this. But, it does come in handy when a person has explosive diarrhea!

Another awkward thing that happened quite often was these were people we knew from our community, which added another layer of discomfort. The day of Cayla's double mastectomy, the medical staff came in to visit, and the main nurse was a guy who served as the music minister at a local church. Not only was he about to see my wife's breasts, but he was going to cut them off! I know these people are medical professionals, but I'm not, and it's a lot to handle the awkwardness of it all.

Navigating disagreements with doctors was another challenge. There were times when Cayla's instincts clashed with the medical advice given, leading to difficult conversations and decisions. One example was when one type of chemo, affectionately and commonly referred to as "the Red Devil," nearly killed her. It took depleted all her white blood cells and left her in the hospital for a week. We decided to end those treatments early. The doctor pushed us to continue, leading to an awkward discussion. Also, her decision to have the double mastectomy and not have reconstructive surgery was often challenged, but we will get into that later on in this book.

Another very important thing I learned through the medical visits process was that often Cayla would not communicate her issues. Cayla is tough and not a complainer at all. But she might have been experiencing fiery diarrhea, and I made it my job to tell on her to the medical staff. Deep down, I think she would admit my candidness with her medical team on her behalf, even to her chagrin, was very helpful. It was crucial for me to advocate for her needs and preferences, even when it was uncomfortable.

Dealing with Sickness and Hospital Stays

Sickness was a constant companion. The treatments caused upset stomachs and, during radiation, Cayla developed sunburn-like symptoms that were incredibly painful. Managing these side effects became a part of our daily routine. I often joked that at my house, we had a fully stocked drug store. If one medicine's side effects made her sick, the answer was always the same: more medicine. We had medicine to offset the negative effects of other medicine.

Hospital stays were particularly challenging. We had two week-long trips to the hospital during her treatments. There's nothing refreshing about sleeping in a hospital as the non-patient. I would go to City Hall during the day and every evening go stay with Cayla at the hospital until the next morning. Get prepared: The machines beep non-stop, and nurses came in at all hours, making it nearly impossible to sleep. I spent many nights on those uncomfortable hospital couches, trying to support Cayla while also dealing with my exhaustion. The lack of privacy and constant interruptions were mentally and physically draining. It's also awkward to be half on and half off that little hospital couch, half dressed, and wake up with a nurse standing right over you.

Awkwardness of Having a Port

One particularly awkward aspect of Cayla's treatment was dealing with her port. The port was necessary for administering medication, but it was a constant reminder of her illness. Now, don't get me wrong, a port is a great medical invention that will save a person from vein blowout, and nothing about vein blowout sounds appealing. Getting the port put in was supposed to be an easy day surgery that somehow resulted in a heart tickle, which put her into AFib, resulting in one of our week-long hospital stays. This got her relationship with her port off on the wrong foot. It seemed to always be sore, and for the first month or two, the nurse accessing the port caused a lot of anxiety for Cayla. She ever so rejoiced the day we had the port removed.

The Fog of "Chemo Brain"

Another significant challenge was the cognitive effects of chemotherapy, often referred to as "chemo brain." For Cayla, it wasn't terrible, but it hit her often. She wouldn't be able to recall things she would normally remember quickly. This would happen and linger for some time after chemo. Most of the time, Cayla would say, "Ahh, chemo brain," and laugh it off, but sometimes it would be very frustrating for her.

Coping with the Awkwardness

Coping with these awkward moments required patience, humor, and a lot of love. We learned to communicate openly about our feelings, even when it was difficult. Finding moments of normalcy and joy amid the chaos was crucial. Whether it was a quick walk, a shared laugh, or simply holding hands, these small acts helped us navigate the awkwardness and stay connected.

We also sought support from our community and leaned on our faith to get through the tough times. Prayer and meditation became essential practices for us, helping to center our minds and find peace amidst the turmoil. Connecting with others who had gone through similar experiences provided us with invaluable insights and a sense of solidarity.

Cancer is a tough road, full of unexpected and often uncomfortable moments. But by facing them together, we found a strength we didn't know we had. Sharing these experiences, as awkward as they were, helped us grow closer and find new ways to love and support each other. I hope that by telling our story, we can help others feel less alone on their journey, and maybe even bring a smile to their faces along the way.

Key Points to Remember During This Time

- ***Dodging Unsolicited Advice:*** Everyone suddenly becomes an expert when cancer's in the picture. From juicing to miracle supplements, you'll hear it all. Smile, nod, and move on.

- ***Hair Today, Gone Tomorrow:*** Watching the locks hit the floor is tough, but sometimes you just have to shave it off and embrace the new look. Sure, it's a tear-jerker, but bald is beautiful. Also, wigs are itchy, hot, and overrated.

- ***Intimacy Interruptus:*** Cancer treatments can really put a damper on the romance. When physical intimacy takes a backseat, get creative with hand-holding, sweet words, and the occasional foot massage. Love finds a way, even if it's not the usual way.

- ***Awkward Medical Moments:*** Nothing says "fun" like a local church music minister/physician's assistant removing your wife's breasts. Stay candid with the doctors, advocate like a professional, and remember everyone's seen worse than whatever awkwardness you're bringing to the table.

Chapter 7: Oh Crap, You Find Out Who Your Friends Are

When you're faced with a life-altering diagnosis like breast cancer, it's as if the whole world gets a magnifying glass held up to it, and you quickly learn the true nature of your friendships. Now, I'll go ahead and say this: not everyone knows how to handle the hardships of others, and that's okay. Even though everywhere I went, all I would hear is, "How's Cayla?" it never got old, because she is my most important person, and it meant a lot that what is important to me was important to other people.

There were people I saw every day, such as at work. They wouldn't ask about it as much as people I might run into at the hardware store, but I knew they cared. They would even say, "I don't ask you about it all the time because I know you probably don't want your mind on it all the time." Now that's a thoughtful approach, and I respected and appreciated it.

Being the mayor of a very small city, I can tell you that the vast majority of people were extremely sympathetic. Some folks in the community didn't even know about it, but it puzzled me how a handful of people that I knew, knew, and they just didn't care. Not one bit. Including this in the book may sound a tad petty, but it's a very true topic. When faced with a major life crisis, you find out who your friends are.

That being said, we had more support than I ever imagined. We had food delivered multiple times a week, which is a very loving gesture, and you remember every person that gave. We had money donated, and you remember every dollar and where it came from. We have a box full of cards with prayers and scripture, and you remember every one of them. They came at such perfect times.

But then there were people who avoided us like we had COVID-19. These people may not have had it in them to lend help, but most seemed just completely selfish. These self-centered people were not strangers. Some were friends, some were coworkers, some were even close family members. They just didn't care. And you remember this. Even now, in this moment, I can still feel it.

The journey is as much about battling the disease as it is about discovering who stands by your side and who quietly fades into the background. This chapter is dedicated to exploring these dynamics and the profound impact they have on your emotional and mental well-being.

True Friends vs. Acquaintances

One of the most startling realizations is differentiating between true friends and mere acquaintances. True friends are those who step up without being asked, offering their time, support, and a listening ear. They check in regularly, bring meals, and sit with you during chemo sessions. We had friends who organized meal trains, helped with the kids, and even sat with Cayla during some of the tougher treatments. Their unwavering support contrasted sharply with others who seemed to disappear when things got tough. Acquaintances, on the other hand, may offer well-meaning but often empty promises. They express sympathy but rarely follow through with meaningful action.

Support in Unexpected Places

Support often comes from the most unexpected places. Coworkers, neighbors, and even strangers can become sources of immense comfort and assistance. The outpouring of kindness from people you barely know can be incredibly moving and restorative. I was amazed by the support from our local community. Neighbors we had only exchanged pleasantries with became pillars of support. Even casual acquaintances at work started checking in on us regularly, offering help in any way they could.

The Role of Long-Term Friends

Long-term friends, with whom you share a deep history, often provide a unique kind of support. Their understanding of your past and shared experiences can be incredibly comforting. These friends bring a sense of normalcy and continuity, reminding you of who you are outside the cancer diagnosis. They knew our history, our quirks, and what would cheer us up. Their visits were like a breath of fresh air, bringing laughter and reminiscing about happier times. Often they would just come and sit. They wouldn't even make us talk, they were just there. It was nice to laugh or hear Cayla laugh. It made a big difference.

Disappointments and Letdowns

It's inevitable that some friends will disappoint you. Whether it's due to their inability to cope with the situation or simply a lack of understanding, these letdowns can be painful. However, understanding and forgiveness are crucial. Not everyone knows how to handle such intense situations, and it's important to recognize that their withdrawal is more about their limitations than a reflection of your worth. We were hurt by a close friend who seemed to vanish when we needed them the most. At first, we felt abandoned and betrayed. Over time, we realized many people struggle with their own issues and simply didn't know how to help. Accepting this helped us let go of the resentment.

Building New Relationships

Facing a crisis can also lead to forming new, meaningful relationships. Support groups and connections with other families dealing with cancer can become invaluable. These new relationships are built on shared experiences and understanding, offering a different kind of comfort. Joining a support group introduced us to families who understood exactly what we were going through. The bond we formed with these new friends was immediate and deep. They became a crucial part of our support network, offering advice, empathy, and companionship. Cayla made a lot of friends by reaching out to other people she knew had cancer. Friends that she still talks to now. It was very often that Cayla would make friends with other patients also. They would even exchange gifts to celebrate each other's milestones.

Maintaining Friendships During Crisis

Maintaining friendships during such a challenging time requires effort and communication. It's essential to articulate your needs clearly and be open to receiving help. Equally important is reciprocating support, ensuring that friendships remain balanced and healthy. We learned to communicate our needs to our friends honestly. Whether it was asking for specific help or simply needing someone to talk to, being open about what we needed made a huge difference. In return, we also made efforts to support our friends, keeping our relationships strong and mutual. It's also noteworthy that some relationships just had to suffer. Our extra needy friends and family relationships suffered the most. We were not emotionally available like normal, but good news! These extra needy friends and family members are still extra needy, even after over a year of our neglect. We were able to pick up the reins of their issues like nothing ever happened.

Key Points to Remember During This Time

- *Appreciate Genuine Support:* Treasure those who show up with a casserole, a kind word, or just their presence. They're the real-life superheroes. It's the lasagna of love that counts, not just the empty words.

- *Understand and Forgive:* Some folks might vanish. It's not you, it's their own hang-ups. So, let it go and save yourself the stress.

- *Communicate Needs Clearly:* People aren't psychic, so don't expect them to be. If you need help, say it loud and clear. "Hey, I need a hand" works wonders compared to silent suffering.

- *Value Unexpected Allies:* Sometimes, support comes from the unlikeliest places. Your chatty neighbor or the coworker you barely know might just be your new best friend. Life's full of surprises.

Chapter 8: Oh Crap, This is Going to Be Bad

As the husband of a wife with breast cancer, the best piece of advice I can give someone else is to take it one day at a time. The journey through cancer treatment is a marathon, not a sprint. When you look at the big picture of all the things you have to go through, it can be majorly overwhelming. Each stage of the process brings its own set of challenges and emotions, and trying to anticipate every twist and turn can quickly lead to feeling overwhelmed. Trust me when I say, breaking it down into manageable steps and focusing on the present moment can make an enormous difference in maintaining your sanity and your wife's morale.

The stress of trying to predict each step can be very overwhelming. Rather than getting bogged down by the 'what-ifs' and the unknowns, try to focus on what you can control: being present, providing support, and taking care of both your physical and emotional needs. Here are a few of our experiences that might help you have a better understanding of what to expect. From dealing with the installation of a port to the harsh realities of chemotherapy and radiation, to coping with unexpected side effects, our journey was a rollercoaster of highs and lows. By sharing these insights, I hope to offer some guidance and reassurance to others walking a similar path. I would like to warn you, don't read all of this and get overwhelmed by it. Just use this section as a reference or maybe even for an, "Yes, we went through this too" moment. If light-hearted and fun is what you are needing, go back and reread the chapter about King Cakes because this isn't the light-hearted and fun part.

Having a Port

When Cayla was told she needed a port, she was understandably nervous. A port is a device implanted under the skin, usually on the right side of the chest, used for drawing blood and administering treatments like chemotherapy, antibiotics, and immunotherapy. It's connected to a catheter that leads to a large vein near the heart. A needle is inserted into the port to deliver treatments or draw blood. The port can stay in place for weeks, months, or even years. The procedure to insert it was supposed to be quick and easy. However, this was not the case for Cayla.

In any medical procedure, there is always a risk. What was supposed to be a quick and easy process turned into an accidental "heart tickle" and a week in the hospital with AFib. I'm not trying to unlock a new level of fears and worry for you; I'm just making the point that you cannot predict a lot of these things. I would also like to add that having a "heart tickle" and AFib is extremely rare and unlikely. Even though we got off to a rocky start, as the treatments progressed, the port became a small blessing in disguise. Instead of enduring constant needle pricks, the port made the process much more bearable. We learned to keep the area clean and watch for any signs of infection, a routine that soon became second nature. We also learned the value of using localized numbing creams, and a lot of it! Over time, the port turned from a source of anxiety into a convenient and essential part of Cayla's treatment.

Chemotherapy and Immunotherapy

Chemotherapy and immunotherapy are words that come with a heavy weight. Chemotherapy uses powerful drugs to kill cancer cells, while immunotherapy boosts the body's immune system to fight the disease. For Cayla, chemotherapy was a tricky experience. The first round that Cayla took was Taxol and Carboplatin. She did this once a week for 12 weeks. It made her hair fall out, and she had to wear ice gloves and socks to help prevent neuropathy. The nausea, fatigue, and hair loss were intense, and there were days when it felt like the treatment was worse than the disease. But this chemo was not impossible to tolerate. The immunotherapy brought its own set of challenges, causing flu-like symptoms, a bad rash in the beginning, and always gave her diarrhea. She did immunotherapy for an entire year. Then the last dose of chemo was Adriamycin, and she was to do a dose every 3 weeks, for 12 weeks. This drug lived up to its name, and the "red devil" nearly killed her by totally zeroing out her white blood cells. This was the cause of her second full week stay in the hospital. Finally, after 2 blood transfusions and 3 different antibiotics, she was able to bounce back. We stopped the "red devil" treatments after her second dose. I told the oncologist he was going to kill her with this "red devil," and he agreed.

Double Mastectomy

Because of the aggressiveness of the cancer Cayla had, removing both breasts to eliminate or reduce the risk of cancer was drastic, but necessary. Surgery day was filled with anxiety, but the procedure went smoothly. The recovery was quicker than we expected. Cayla managed the pain with prescribed medications and the support of a strong network of family, friends, and a nice lift chair my parents bought her. We focused on following the doctor's post-operative instructions, and I learned how to empty post-surgical drain bags. It was weird seeing her go into surgery with triple D breasts and coming out, an hour later, flat as a board. The best news was, they removed everything, tested it all, and there was no sign of cancer.

Radiation

Radiation therapy, intended to kill any remaining cancerous cells, was another daunting part of the journey. The oncologist explained it like this: you have cancer, we are going to shrink the cancer with chemo and boost your immune system with immunotherapy. Then the surgeon will remove all the tumors. Then the radiation will be administered to catch any speck of cancer dust that might be floating around in there.

Cayla had to undergo 33 radiation treatments. Because of her age, they opted for a type of radiation called proton radiation, which allowed them to focus on the troubled areas without accidentally damaging surrounding organs. We had heard mixed experiences about it, but nothing prepared us for the severity of Cayla's reaction. Her light, white skin turned pink, then red, then dark red, then dark brown like very dark leather. She was sore and blistered, making the daily treatments increasingly painful. The actual daily treatments were mostly easy, quick, and painless. But the ongoing burning of the skin was painful. We took it one session at a time, focusing on the end goal of beating the cancer.

Strange Side Effects

Cancer treatments often come with a host of unexpected side effects that can significantly impact daily life. While some side effects are well-known, others can catch you off guard and add layers of complexity to an already challenging journey. Here are some of the strange side effects we encountered during Cayla's treatment and how we managed to cope with them.

Chemotherapy caused Cayla's nails to become brittle and break easily. Chemotherapy can make nails weak and brittle. They may even start to split from the tissue holding them in place, a condition known as onycholysis. In some cases, nails might fall off after several rounds of treatment. Certain chemotherapy drugs, like Taxol and Taxotere, are more likely to cause nail loss than others. It was surprising how such a small detail could cause so much discomfort and fear. We found that keeping her nails short so they would not get caught on anything and moisturized helped reduce the breakage and associated pain. She would also keep a clear coat of fingernail polish on them to give them a little strength. By babying them, she was able to avoid losing any nails.

Thanks to her medication such as her antiviral, her skin became extremely sensitive, burning easily even with minimal sun exposure. This was a drastic change from her pre-treatment days when she could spend time outdoors without any issues. Tanning, something she used to enjoy, was out of the question.

After the removal of lymph nodes, Cayla experienced lymphedema, which caused her arm to swell. Managing this swelling requires her to wear a compression sleeve, an added inconvenience that she had to incorporate into her daily routine. The sleeve helps control the swelling, but it is a constant reminder of the physical changes brought on by her treatment. When Cayla realized she would need to do this every day from now on, she was devastated. She resented the idea of wearing that sleeve, "like an old lady." Out of everything, she seemed to take this the hardest, which in typical male fashion, I did not understand. I understand it more now because it is a lifelong sentence. Her eyebrows and hair will grow back, but that sleeve is an everyday, unwelcome companion. But, she realizes that the alternative of not wearing that sleeve is worse. She even has a sleeve that looks like a full arm tattoo sleeve. She's made the best out of the situation.

One of the most challenging side effects was the early onset of menopause induced by the treatments, leading to frequent and intense hot flashes. These hot flashes are not just uncomfortable; they are a stark reminder of the hormonal upheaval her body was undergoing. Cayla still has hot flashes, and does not like to get real hot, but she manages it still with medications and courage.

Another unexpected side effect was muscle, bone, and joint pain. All of a sudden, my 36-year-old wife was walking around like an elderly grandma, especially in the mornings. The stiffness and discomfort were most pronounced after periods of rest, making it difficult for her to start the day. We bought a nice handheld massager that seemed to help a lot. This added yet another layer of complexity to her daily life, but we managed to find ways to ease the pain through gentle exercises, stretching, and medication

Key Points to Remember During This Time

- *Pace Yourself:* The road ahead is long and winding. Focus on each mile marker instead of the whole route. Small victories add up, keeping you and your wife grounded.
- *Stay Flexible:* Cancer treatment has its own twists and turns. Be prepared to get thrown some curve balls. It's part of it.
- *Master the Mundane:* While you can't foresee every challenge, you can nail the everyday stuff. Keep the ship steady by taking care of the basics—support, self-care, and staying present. Consistency is your secret weapon.
- *Embrace the Beautiful Mess:* Life's about to get messy, and that's perfectly fine. Accept the chaos and roll with it.

Chapter 9: Oh Crap, Battling the Blues

Navigating through a loved one's cancer journey can be emotionally exhausting, and it's natural to feel the weight of the world on your shoulders. In this chapter, we'll explore ways to combat the emotional lows and maintain a positive outlook even in the face of adversity.

Defeating Worry by Reverse Worrying

One effective way to manage worry is by practicing reverse worrying. Instead of fixating on what could go wrong, shift your focus to what could go right. This technique involves actively visualizing positive outcomes and successes.

When Cayla was going through her treatment, I found myself worrying about the worst-case scenarios. It was consuming and exhausting. We've all heard advice like "just stop worrying" or "why worry, it does no good." We also know that worry is extremely powerful, backed by strong emotions and intense focus. Telling someone to just stop worrying is like telling a cow to stop eating the grass in the field or asking a tree not to move when the wind blows. It can't be done. I'm going to worry. You are going to worry too.

One day, I decided to try something different. Instead of thinking about all the things that could go wrong, I started visualizing everything that could go right. I imagined Cayla finishing her treatment successfully, our family celebrating the end of her chemotherapy, and her health gradually improving. I saw successful, happy endings before they ever happened, and then I saw them again in our reality. This shift in mindset was incredibly powerful. It didn't eliminate the challenges, but it helped me see the possibilities and stay hopeful.

I tried it on other things too. I would find myself saying, "What if I don't have enough money to make it until the next payday?" I would change it to "What if I have enough money to make it?" When I thought, "What if a bill comes in that I can't pay?" I would change it to "What if money comes in that I'm not expecting?" When I worried, "What if she gets a bad report?" I would change it to "What if we get great news today?" Try this technique. Something about it will make you nearly instantly feel better.

They say that over 80% of the things people worry about never come true. So why not worry about something good happening? The mind needs something to do. Feed it something that will benefit you and your family.

To practice reverse worrying, take a few moments each day to close your eyes and imagine positive scenarios. What's bothering you? Reverse it. See yourself and your loved one overcoming challenges and celebrating victories. Write down a list of potential successes, no matter how small. It could be a successful doctor's visit, a day without pain, or simply a moment of joy. Celebrate these small achievements, as each small win can build momentum and foster a positive mindset.

Gratitude and Fear Can't Coexist

Gratitude is a powerful antidote to fear and anxiety. When you focus on what you're thankful for, it's difficult for fear to take hold. Practicing daily gratitude can help you stay grounded and positive. Have you ever been thankful? Sure you have. Have you ever been worried badly? Sure you have. But have you ever been in a state of gratitude and a state of worry at the same time? No, those two emotional levels can't coexist.

Cayla has always been good at reminding me to see the positive things in my life. There really is always something to be thankful for. Family, friends, community, our jobs, homes, possessions. If you are spiraling into depression or fear, I have hard news to tell you: you've gotten too self-focused. Turn your focus inside out and start counting your blessings.

Positive Self Talk

There were times when Cayla would get very depressed. Thankfully, these times didn't last long, and considering all she went through, they were not very frequent. Dr. Shad Helmstetter wrote a book called "What to Say When You Talk to Yourself." It's an awesome book about the power of what we are saying to ourselves. He also has an app that you can subscribe to that will speak positive and powerful sentences to you. On days when Cayla got really down or upset, I would encourage her to lay down and listen to her self-talk recordings. The recordings that she liked were called "Quality of Life." Within minutes, her spirit and energy would be lifted back up to a manageable and normal level.

The Power of Faith

Faith is the most underrated and the biggest hidden key to life there is. Throughout our journey, our medical doctors and surgeons often gave us advice like, "This treatment will work if you stay positive." It was said in different ways, such as, "The medicine will work, but you also can't get depressed," or "You have to push for a successful treatment." All these are, in essence, saying, "According to your faith, it will be done."

People would tell me they were praying. I feel like it's important to tell people what to pray for, so that's what I would do. I did not want people praying these kinds of prayers: "Poor Cayla, don't let her die," or "Be with this family, they are struggling." No, I wanted prayers like, "Cayla is having surgery tomorrow. Let it be successful," or "Cayla is in the hospital with low white blood cell counts; please pray that her counts would go up." This is the way to be prayed for. Direct everyone's attention. All that positivity is faith, and faith really makes all the difference.

Spend time visualizing the outcomes you want to achieve. This helps in creating a mental roadmap to guide your actions. I have learned in my life that God is absolutely faithful to our specific requests. Visualization of success coupled with the belief that success will be is the key to that faith.

Compartmentalizing

While we discussed compartmentalizing in a previous chapter, it's worth revisiting briefly. Compartmentalizing can help you manage overwhelming emotions by breaking down problems into manageable parts.

I often found myself overwhelmed by the sheer volume of challenges we faced. Compartmentalizing became a lifesaver. I learned to break down larger issues into smaller, more manageable tasks. Instead of trying to tackle everything at once, I focused on one task at a time. This approach helped me stay organized and less overwhelmed.

Prioritizing tasks became essential for me. I learned to identify the most critical tasks and focus on them first. Letting go of less important tasks that could wait was difficult but necessary. Taking regular breaks and practicing mindfulness also made a significant difference. Even a few minutes of deep breathing or a short walk outside helped me reset and recharge.

Not only did I compartmentalize to divide issues into manageable pieces, but I also compartmentalized by letting go of the situation at times. For example, when I was at City Hall, I would deal with city issues. When I was at home, I would deal with home issues. When I was accompanying Cayla to the doctor, I would be all in at the doctor.

The Importance of Positive Energy

As a couple, you feed off each other's energy. It's essential to keep your energy up, not by faking it or being an eternal optimist out of touch with reality, but by maintaining a balanced emotional state. Getting depressed yourself is not going to help your spouse. Have your moments, and then get yourself back to an emotional level where both you and your spouse can move forward.

When I felt down, I realized that Cayla could sense it, and it affected her mood as well. It's not about putting on a fake smile, but about finding genuine ways to lift your spirits so that you can be a source of strength for each other. Take time for self-care, seek support from friends or a counselor, and engage in activities that bring you joy. This balance will help both of you navigate the journey with more resilience.

Key Points to Remember During This Time

- *Use positive self-talk like:* "We've got this!"
- *Flip the Script on Worry:* Instead of dwelling on doom and gloom, visualize everything going right.
- *Faith is Your Superpower:* Trust in the power of faith to guide you through tough times. Direct prayers and positive energy towards specific outcomes, and believe that good things are on the horizon.
- *Master the Art of Compartmentalizing:* Tackle problems one piece at a time. Focus on the task at hand.
- *When All Else Fails:* Go get some king cake!

Chapter 10: Oh Crap, She Said 'Off with Her Boobs'

Cayla faced a monumental decision in her breast cancer journey: opting for a double mastectomy and deciding against any reconstructive surgery. This choice surprised many, including her doctor, who initially believed she would change her mind and recommended the most renowned reconstructive surgeon in the state.

Research and Considerations

Cayla's decision was not made lightly. She spent countless hours researching various reconstruction options:

1. DIEP Flap Surgery: This procedure involves using tissue from the lower abdomen to recreate the breast mound. It spares the abdominal muscles, which can reduce recovery time and maintain abdominal strength, but it is complex and involves a significant recovery period.

2. Implant Reconstruction: This involves inserting silicone or saline-filled prostheses to recreate the breast shape. A critical step in this process often involves the use of skin expanders. These are temporary, balloon-like devices inserted under the skin and chest muscle. Over several weeks or months, these expanders are gradually filled with saline solution, stretching the skin to create enough space for the final implant. However, this process can be uncomfortable and requires multiple visits

to the surgeon.

3. Autologous Fat Transfer: This method involves liposuctioning fat from other parts of the body and injecting it into the breast area. While it can produce a very natural feel, it often requires multiple sessions and can result in fat necrosis, where the transferred fat cells die and form hard lumps.

4. The Goldilocks Procedure: Due to radiation treatments, Cayla considered this innovative technique. It involves rearranging the remaining breast tissue and skin after a mastectomy to create a breast mound that can be left as is or later augmented with implants or fat grafting. This procedure can provide a natural contour and shape but also involves its own set of challenges and recovery.

Conversations with friends who had faced complications from reconstructive surgeries further solidified Cayla's resolve. Stories of implants shifting, capsular contracture, and multiple corrective surgeries made her cautious.

One friend shared her experience of implants shifting out of position, which required several surgeries to correct. Each surgery brought with it a new set of challenges and recovery periods, disrupting her life significantly. The constant adjustments and the physical pain were not something Cayla wanted to endure.

Another friend spoke about capsular contracture, where scar tissue forms tightly around the implant, causing hardness and discomfort. This condition often necessitates additional surgeries to remove or replace the implants. The thought of facing such complications made Cayla wary of the long-term implications of reconstructive surgery.

Lastly, Cayla heard about the emotional toll multiple corrective surgeries took on her friends. Each procedure brought anxiety, uncertainty, and frustration. The prospect of enduring ongoing medical interventions, with no guarantee of a satisfactory outcome, convinced

Cayla that her decision to go flat and avoid reconstruction was the best choice for her peace of mind and well-being.

Cayla's Decision Process

The pivotal moment came during a consultation with her doctor. As he detailed the reconstruction techniques, recovery times, potential complications, and aesthetic outcomes, Cayla listened intently. When he finished, she calmly said, "No, I'm not doing any of that. I'm going flat."

At home, our conversations about this decision were heartfelt and honest. I expressed my concerns and fears that she might regret it later. However, Cayla reassured me with unwavering confidence. She felt more in control of her body and life by making this decision, wanting to avoid further surgeries, pain, and uncertainty.

Life After the Decision

Cayla embraced her choice with the same courage that saw her through chemotherapy, where she proudly rocked her bald head. She found a supportive online community through YouTube and TikTok, gaining practical advice and emotional support from others who had made similar choices.

In public, Cayla wears prosthetic breasts. With a shirt on, you would never know the difference. These prosthetics allow her to feel comfortable and confident in her appearance. At home, she often goes without them, embracing her natural form.

Emotional Journey

My initial mixed feelings gradually changed. Seeing her without a top took some getting used to, but I realized that breasts did not define her or our relationship. Cayla had been through enough, and additional surgeries seemed unnecessary. Her strength and resilience have been nothing short of inspiring, showing everyone that true beauty and strength come from within.

One of the most touching aspects of this journey has been witnessing Cayla's interactions with other women facing similar decisions. She has become a source of support and inspiration, sharing her story openly and helping others navigate the challenging terrain of breast cancer.

Cayla's decision to go flat and stay flat is a testament to her inner strength and commitment to living life on her own terms. It's a powerful reminder that our bodies are just one part of who we are, and true beauty comes from within. As we move forward together, I am more inspired than ever by her courage and resilience. She is, and always will be, my hero.

And hey, her prosthetics have added a bit of fun to our lives. Sometimes, I'll jokingly ask, "Are we going for the low-key look tonight or can you bring out the big ones?" Cayla will usually roll her eyes and wear them. Occasionally, I tease her about leaving her boobs on the bathroom counter. To be completely honest, it's not been that bad. These light-hearted moments help us stay connected and keep a sense of humor through it all.

Key Points to Remember During This Time

- *Support and Communication:* Open, honest communication with your partner is crucial. Discuss your concerns, fears, and thoughts openly to support each other emotionally.
- *Respect Individual Decisions:* Understand and respect your partner's choices regarding their body and treatment options. Recognize that these decisions are deeply personal and should be supported.
- *Focus on Practical Needs:* Stay organized with medical appointments, treatments, and medications. Keep a calendar or planner to track important dates and tasks. Ensure a comfortable and supportive home environment to aid in recovery and emotional well-being.
- *Maintain a Sense of Humor:* Find moments of lightness and humor in your daily life. This can be a powerful tool to cope with stress and maintain a positive outlook.
- *Engage in activities*: that bring joy and laughter, helping to strengthen your bond and create cherished memories.

Chapter 11: Oh Crap, Life Moves On

Life Moves On for Cayla

Cayla's experience post-cancer has been a journey of adaptation and resilience. While the treatments and surgeries have ended, the physical and emotional impacts continue to shape her daily life. This section delves into the various ways Cayla has navigated the aftermath of cancer, highlighting her ongoing challenges and personal growth.

Physical and Medical Adjustments

Cayla's journey through breast cancer was grueling, but the aftermath brought its own set of challenges. One of the biggest shocks for her was the necessity of wearing a compression sleeve to manage lymphedema. I never expected that a simple piece of clothing could have such a significant impact on her daily life. She eventually accepted this new reality and has learned to incorporate the sleeve into her routine faithfully.

Another thing that has taken us both by surprise is that regular check-ups with her oncologist have become a source of anxiety. I could tell that she gets very anxious the closer we get to her follow-up appointments. We had a long discussion about it, and she explained that since she has been declared with no sign of cancer, she has moved on from being a patient to being a regular person again. But periodically, she has to go back to her oncologist for a follow-up appointment. Each appointment feels like stepping back into the role of a patient, which is difficult after trying so hard to reclaim a sense of normalcy.

She also still has some minor issues from radiation. For example, she has to massage the areas where she received radiation treatments, a constant reminder of the battle she fought. Persistent hot flashes, though regulated by medication, still disrupt her life and serve as another lingering side effect of the treatment.

Survivor's Guilt and Fear of Recurrence

Being declared cancer-free was a moment of immense relief for Cayla. We threw a party at our house and invited many people who supported us through the journey. She rung the bell on her last day of chemotherapy and took pictures wearing a custom shirt that said, "Last day of radiation," on her final day of treatment. To celebrate her last days with her breasts, we went on a special trip we called "Ta-Ta to the Tatas." It was a joyous victory, but it also brought an unexpected emotional burden: survivor's guilt.

She often struggled with the reality that while she could celebrate her victories, there were countless others still fighting for their lives. Every time we celebrated her victories, there was a nagging reminder that others were still in the midst of their battles. For every milestone we reached, someone else was facing setbacks and uncertainties. This mix of joy for our progress and sorrow for others created a tough emotional balance. We felt incredibly blessed, but at the same time, our hearts ached for those still suffering.

This guilt is compounded by the fear of recurrence. Despite her double mastectomy, she remains vigilant, performing self-checks and monitoring areas like her underarms and neck where lymph nodes are located. Every ache or unusual feeling can trigger a wave of anxiety, bringing back memories of the initial diagnosis and the uncertainty that followed. The anxiety of what might be lurking beneath the surface never fully dissipates; it's a shadow that follows her, a constant reminder of the fragility of remission. She is on a check-up schedule that includes regular blood work and doctor visits for the rest of her life, so we really shouldn't worry. But it's always in the back of your mind—a bit of PTSD probably.

Hair Styles and Clothing Differences

One of the more visible changes has been her hair. Growing it back to almost shoulder length has been a journey in itself, filled with challenges. The process was slow and often frustrating, as she watched her hair gradually return. There were days when it seemed like no progress was being made, and the uneven growth required constant attention. Despite these difficulties, reaching the milestone of shoulder-length hair has been a significant achievement.

To help with the regrowth process, Cayla has had to use extensions to fill in gaps and add length where needed. These extensions have not only helped with the aesthetics but have also provided a boost to her confidence. Embracing her natural salt-and-pepper hair has been empowering. She made the decision to forego coloring and embrace the natural changes, which has led to an unexpected benefit—she now receives compliments on her hair every day. This shift in her appearance has become a source of pride and a symbol of her resilience.

Adjusting to clothes fitting differently has also been part of this new reality. The fake breasts, though necessary, are not always comfortable and have significantly changed how her clothes fit and feel on her body. Shopping for clothes that accommodate the changes has been a challenging task. She often finds herself needing to buy new items that provide both comfort and style. The physical discomfort and the psychological adjustment to her new body image have been ongoing struggles, but they are also a testament to her strength and adaptability in the face of profound change.

Public Perception and Personal Growth

People often expect Cayla to bounce back and be her old self, but the truth is, she's a new person now. The journey through breast cancer has fundamentally changed her. Her priorities have shifted dramatically, with a newfound emphasis on what truly matters in life. The experience has deepened her perspective, making her more reflective and appreciative of the small moments. This growth is something she cherishes, even if it means not meeting others' expectations of who she should be.

Living with this new reality, Cayla has learned to navigate the delicate balance between honoring her personal growth and managing the expectations of those around her. Some people struggle to understand why she isn't the same person she was before her diagnosis, but she has come to accept that their perspective is limited by their lack of firsthand experience. This acceptance has empowered her to focus on her own journey and the lessons she has learned along the way.

Speaking at a breast cancer fundraiser was a significant milestone in her journey. Addressing a room of 200 people, she shared her story and advocated for awareness. It was an emotional experience, filled with both tears and triumphs, but it also felt like a powerful way for her to give back and support others facing similar battles. Through her speech, Cayla was able to connect with others on a deep level, offering them hope and solidarity. This opportunity to advocate and share her journey publicly has reinforced her sense of purpose and commitment to helping others navigate their own battles with cancer.

Life Moves On for Nick

My journey alongside Cayla has led to profound changes and realizations. From handling the stress of her illness to finding new ways to support others, I've learned invaluable lessons. This chapter details our experiences and the strategies we've developed to turn our challenges into sources of strength and inspiration for others.

Financial and Career Adjustments

We had a small cancer policy, but the financial hit was still significant. My business, which Cayla was going to run, suffered. As a further blow, my key employee passed away suddenly, which was devastating. Financially, it's been hard to get back on track. However, Cayla has a new job at our local courthouse, and she's doing well.

Changes in Appearance and Acceptance

Cayla has always been beautiful, even when she had no hair or eyebrows. But I'm really enjoying the fact that she has hair again. I've even grown to like her fake eyelashes. I used to love her nearly black hair, but now it's a salt-and-pepper color, which I've come to appreciate. It shows that we've been through a lot together.

I've been eating healthier all year, resulting in significant weight loss. I'm not where I want to be yet, but I'm headed in the right direction. Cayla seems more content in life than ever, and I'm so proud of that. She used to serve others so hard, almost as if to win their affection. Pre-cancer, I would tell her that she is so amazing, she doesn't have to do everything she does. Now, she seems very content and self-confident. That's an unexpected consequence of our journey. Through the love and support shown during cancer, I feel more accepted, and it has made me a more confident mayor.

Embracing Simplicity and New Routines

We've planted a garden in an effort to enjoy simpler things while eating better. The first thing we do in the morning is make a pot of coffee and then check our garden. We've really enjoyed it. Cayla can swim again, something she couldn't do at all last year. Rebuilding wasn't instant, but we have gotten back to a pretty normal life again.

Coping with Stress and Anxiety

The times that Cayla has stress and anxiety have surprised me. I really thought she wouldn't be anxious anymore. But I find that being with her really helps. I take time off to go to her appointments and still tell her doctor about her issues because she isn't always fully transparent. When Cayla is really stressed, I put on bluegrass music. It oddly calms her down, though I must warn, it probably won't work on most ladies.

Changes in Our Love Life

Due to all the changes in her body, our love life has changed. It's not nonexistent, but it's not like it was. The good news is I turned 40 somewhere in the middle of this journey, and I don't know if it's being over 40 or just life in general, but I don't really care. I'm just glad she's here.

over 40 or just life in general, but I don't really care. I'm just glad she's here.

Key Points to Remember During This Time

- ***Adapting to Changes:*** Nothing is the same, and you won't even be the same. A cancer survivor goes through so much; you won't be the same, and you probably will not look the same. Embrace it. It's a new chapter, and there is still a lot of life to live.
- ***Managing Survivor's Guilt:*** Celebrate your victories without holding back. It's also okay to care about others who are struggling.
- ***Turn Ashes into Victory:*** Once this is over, you will have lived through a life lesson that compares to no other. Don't miss your successes just because they were hard experiences.
- ***Spouses Change Too:*** The spouse of a cancer survivor won't ever be the same either. This journey changes both partners, bringing new perspectives and challenges. Embrace these changes and grow together.

Closing Remarks

Thank you for taking the time to read our story and for joining us on this journey. We hope that the experiences we've shared have provided you with valuable insights and support as you navigate your own challenges. Remember, you are not alone, and there is strength in community.

If you found this content helpful, we invite you to stay connected and receive updates, tips, and additional resources by signing up for our email alerts. By subscribing, you'll be the first to know about new content, upcoming events, and exclusive offers.

Join our community today and stay informed:

For more information or support, please visit us at https://www.ohcrapbreastcancer.com/signup or check out our YouTube channel at https://www.youtube.com/@NickCayla.

We appreciate your support and look forward to continuing this journey together.

Warm regards,

Nick and Cayla Cox

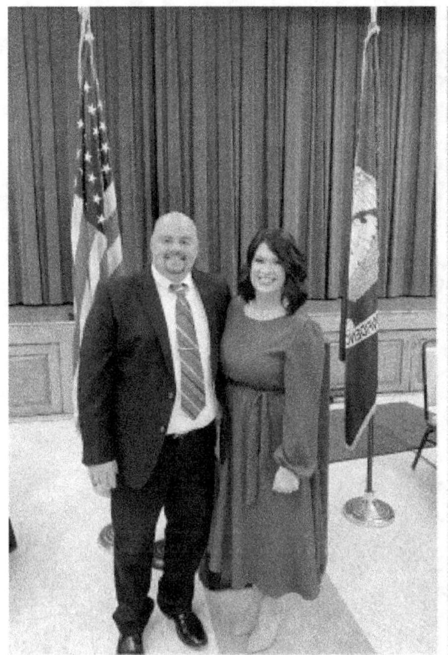

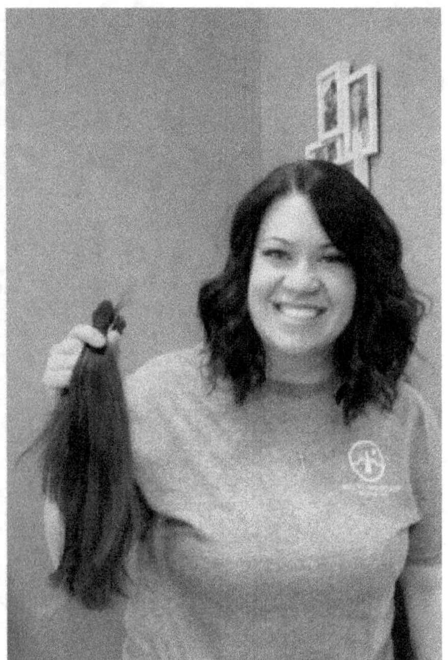

"You have breast cancer" words we never wanted to hear and absolutely did not see on the horizon for 2023. Please pray for Cayla Cox and our family as we spend this year getting her cancer free. She starts Tuesday with 24 weeks of chemo. We are so thankful and blessed to be surrounded with a community of prayer warriors and caring people. We are people of faith and our hope is in the Lord.

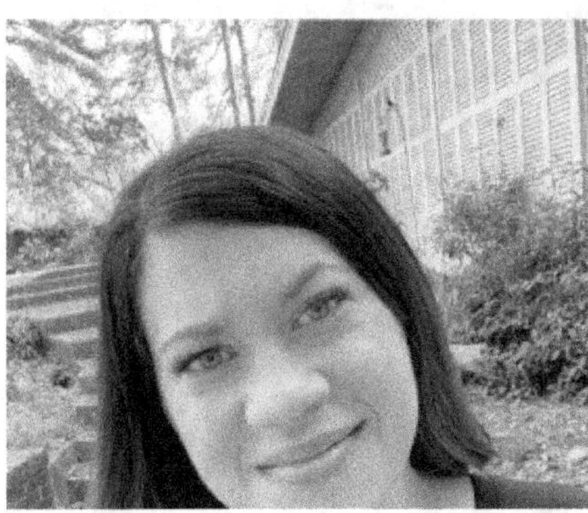

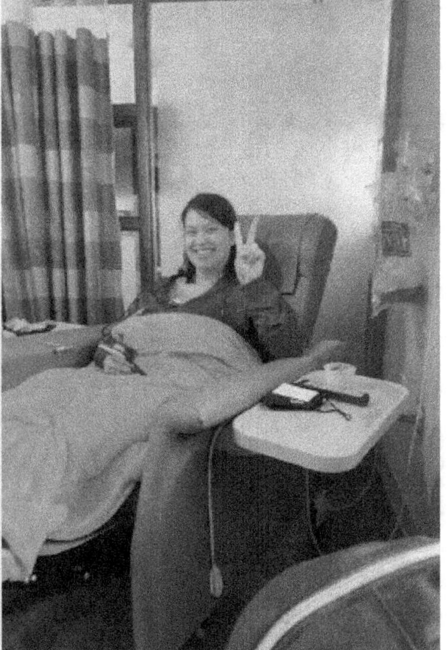

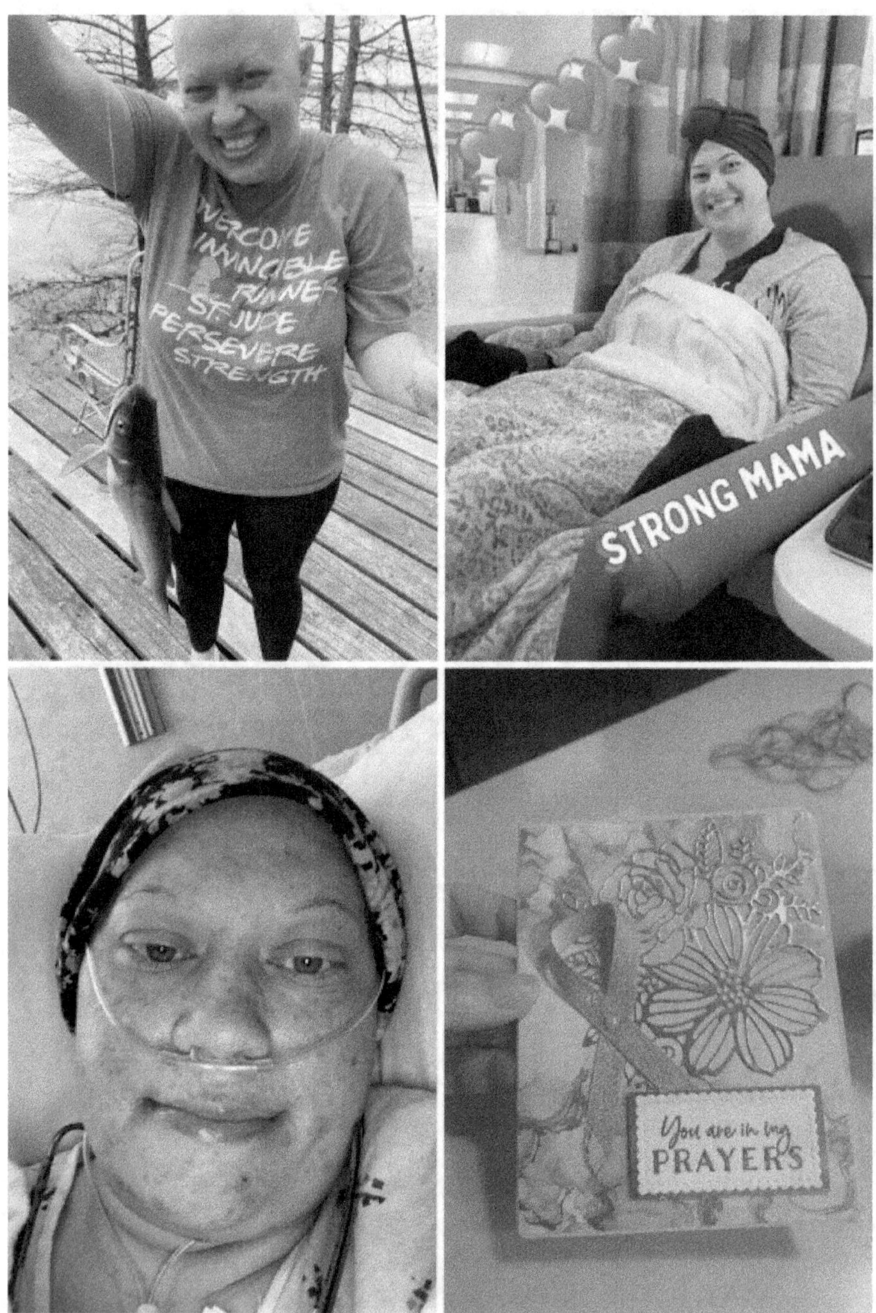
OVERCOME
INVINCIBLE
RUNNER
ST JUDE
PERSEVERE
STRENGTH
STRONG MAMA
You are in my
PRAYERS

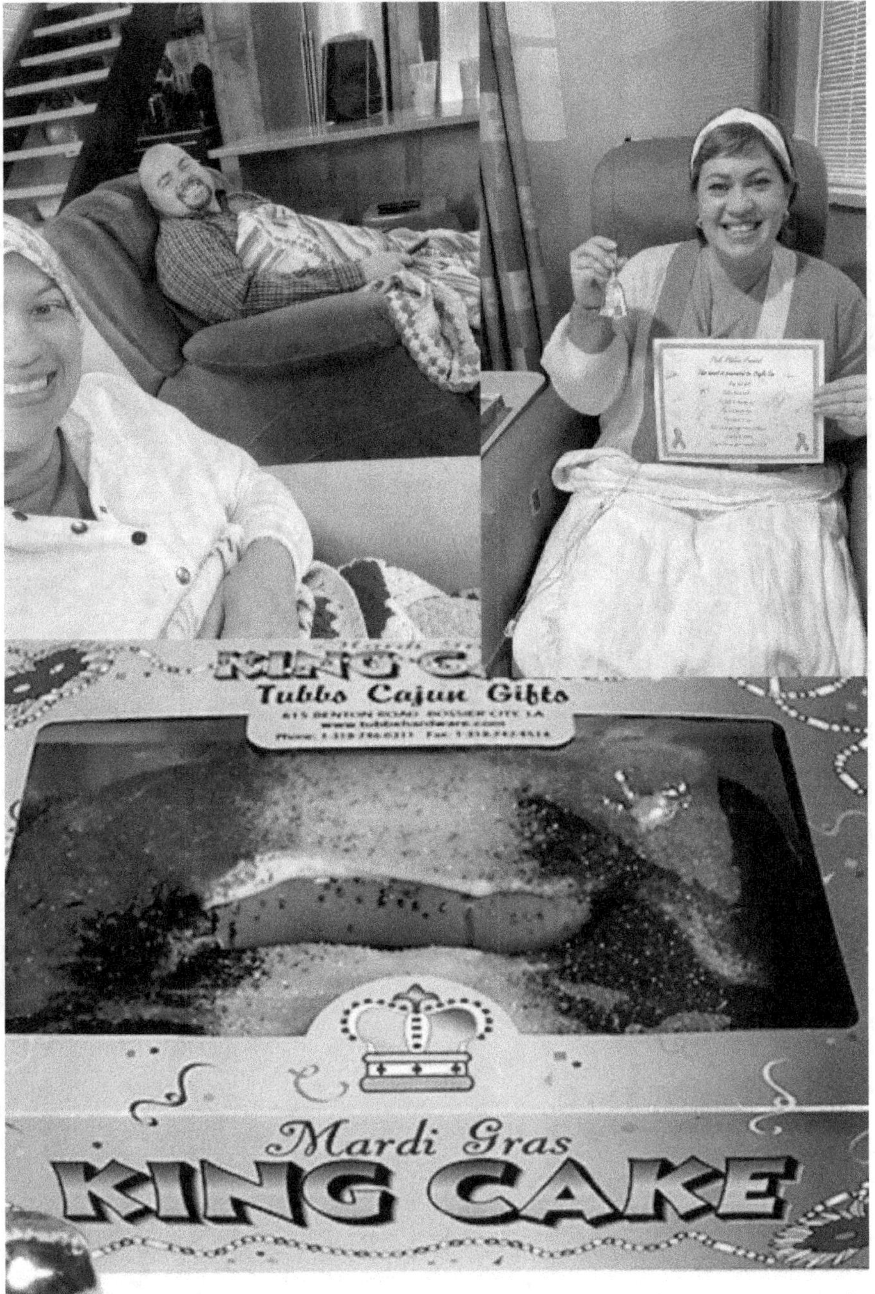
Tubbs Cajun Gifts
Mardi Gras
KING CAKE

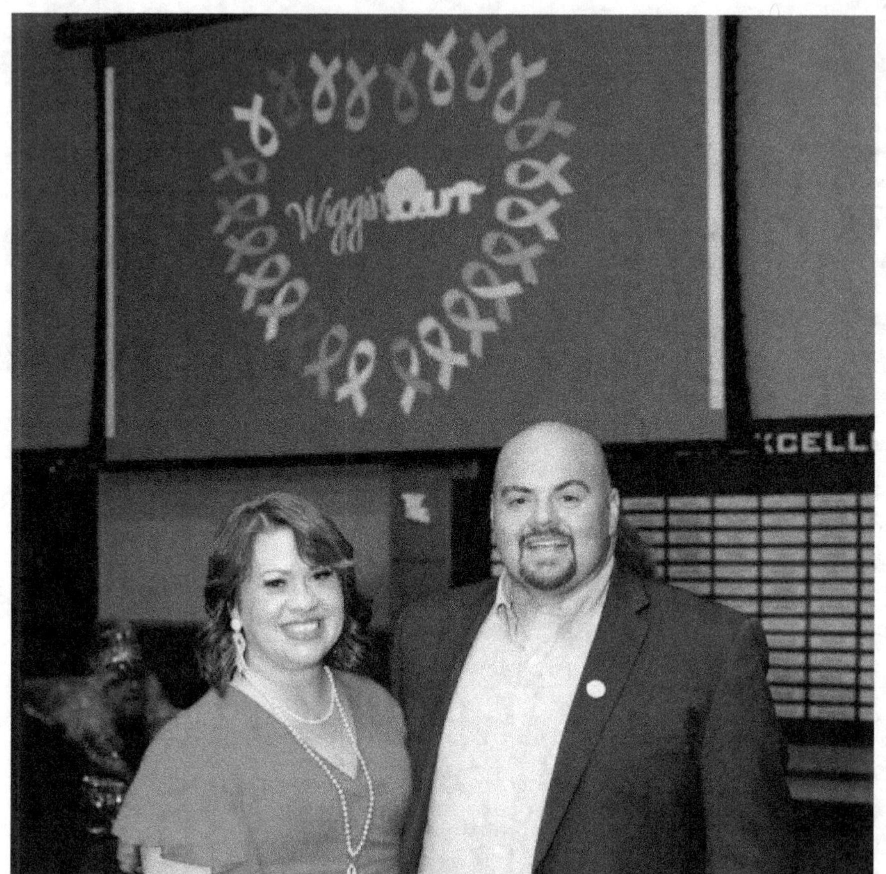
Wiggin OUT

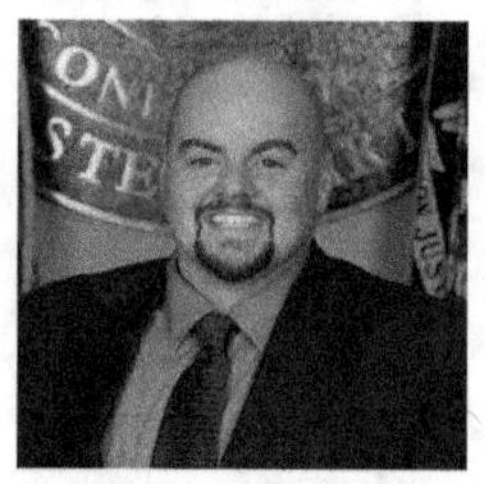

About the Author

Nick Cox is the mayor The City of Minden, of a small city in north Louisiana and a dedicated husband and father. When his wife, Cayla, was diagnosed with stage 3 breast cancer, Nick found himself navigating the dual challenges of public service and personal crisis. Drawing from his experiences, Nick shares his journey to offer support and guidance to other husbands and partners facing similar battles. His writing is marked by honesty, resilience, and a touch of humor, reflecting his belief in the power of love and community. Nick is committed to helping couples find strength and hope during their toughest times.

Read more at https://www.ohcrapbreastcancer.com/.

www.ingramcontent.com/pod-product-compliance
Lightning Source LLC
Chambersburg PA
CBHW072032150726
47999CB00002B/860